PILATES FOR BEGINNERS

The Essential Guide for Total Body Fitness, Strong Muscles and Lean Body (A Manual for Beginners)

Andrew Schwarzenegger

Table of Contents

CHAPTER ONE

What is Pilates?

Pilates is a kind of exercise that aims to strengthen muscles while improving postural alignment and flexibility. Joseph Pilates developed it in the early twentieth century, originally as a rehabilitation program for prisoners of war. Pilates felt that mental and physical health were inextricably linked, and his program emphasized core strength, balance, and coordination.

Pilates concepts include the following

Pilates movements emphasis on the core muscles of the belly, lower back, hips, and buttocks.

Concentration: Practitioners are advised to concentrate on the movements they are doing to ensure perfect form and technique.

Pilates movements are performed with control and accuracy, rather than velocity.

Precision: Each Pilates action has a defined function and is executed with meticulous attention to detail.

Breath: Pilates requires proper breathing, with intake and exhalation timed with activity.

Pilates movements are designed to flow seamlessly from one to the next, instilling a feeling of grace and fluidity.

The benefits of Pilates for beginners include

Pilates focuses on strengthening the core muscles, which may help with stability and posture.

Stretching is often used in Pilates exercises to increase flexibility and range of motion.

Better posture: Pilates may help address postural abnormalities, resulting in improved alignment and reduced strain on the body.

Pilates promotes attentive movement, which may increase body awareness and coordination.

Pilates, by increasing core strength and posture, may help lower the chance of injury during athletic activity.

Stress relief: Pilates, like other types of exercise, may help relieve stress and enhance mental health.

Overall, Pilates is a mild yet effective kind of exercise that may help beginners improve strength, flexibility, posture, and body awareness.

Prepare for your first Pilates session.

Preparing for your first Pilates lesson will help you feel more at ease and maximize the benefits of your exercise. Here's everything you'll need:

Essential Equipment:

A Pilates or yoga mat offers padding and traction for floor-based workouts.

Resistance bands may be used to increase resistance and strength during workouts.

The Pilates Ring, also known as the Magic Circle, is a flexible ring used to provide resistance to arm and leg workouts.

Small Pilates Ball: This is useful for workouts that target particular muscles, such as the inner thighs or abdominals.

Clothing:

Wear comfortable, form-fitting clothes that enables you to move about easily.

Avoid wearing too baggy apparel that might get in the way or get tangled during exercise.

Footwear:

Pilates is usually performed barefoot or with grip socks to avoid sliding on the mat.

If you choose to wear shoes, go for lightweight, flexible shoes with adequate grip.

Stay hydrated throughout your exercise by keeping a water bottle handy.

Towel: Keep a towel nearby to wipe away perspiration and offer extra cushioning if necessary.

Creating a suitable workout space

Choose a calm, well-ventilated environment with plenty of space to walk about.

Remove any impediments or distractions that might interfere with your training.

If feasible, set aside a distinct place for your Pilates practice to establish a consistent and welcoming environment.

By preparing these necessities and creating an appropriate training environment, you can make the most of your first Pilates session and set yourself up for a successful and fun workout.

CHAPTER TWO

Key Pilates exercises

The Hundred: Lie on your back, raise your legs to a tabletop posture, then elevate your head and shoulders off the mat. Pump your arms up and down while inhaling and exhaling for five counts each, for a total of 100 pumps.

The Roll-Up: Lie on your back, arms extended above. Exhale as you pull your spine off the mat and stretch forward to touch your toes. Inhale and roll back down with control.

The Single Leg Stretch: Lie on your back, knees bent, and shins parallel to the ground. Bring one knee in towards your chest while extending the other leg out. Switch legs in a scissor-like action while lifting your head and shoulders off the mat.

The Double Leg Stretch begins in the same posture as the Single Leg Stretch. Bring both knees in to your chest, then extend both legs at a 45-degree angle. Circle your arms around to hug your knees back in while maintaining your head and shoulders up.

The Plank: Begin in a push-up posture, hands squarely beneath your shoulders. Engage your core and straighten your legs, keeping a straight line from head to heels.

Pilates Breathing Techniques
Pilates stresses lateral breathing, which involves inhaling through

your nose and expanding your ribcage to the sides and back, enabling the lungs to fill completely.

Exhale through your lips, bringing your navel toward your spine to activate your deep core muscles.

Proper alignment and posture

Maintain a neutral spine by retaining your lower back's natural curvature without arching or flattening it.

Draw your navel towards your spine and elevate your pelvic floor to engage your core muscles.

Maintain a comfortable posture with shoulders away from your ears and a long neck.

Align your limbs and joints correctly to avoid tension and optimize the efficacy of each exercise.

These fundamental Pilates exercises, breathing methods, and concepts of appropriate alignment and posture are essential for a safe and efficient Pilates practice.

Structure a Beginner-Friendly Pilates Workout

Warm-up (5 to 10 minutes):

Begin by warming up your body with moderate motions like walking in place, shoulder rolls, and spinal twists.

Incorporate breathing exercises to help you focus and connect with your breath.

Main Workout: (20-30 minutes)

Start with core-focused exercises like the Hundred, Roll-Up, and Single Leg Stretch.

Move on to movements that target other regions of the body, such as the legs, arms, and back, while keeping the core engaged.

Cool-down (5–10 minutes):

Gently stretch the muscles used in the exercise, concentrating on the hamstrings, hips, back, and shoulders.

Finish with relaxation activities, such as deep breathing or a short meditation, to promote peace and well-being.

Progressing Safely in Your Practice

Listen to Your Body: Notice how your body feels during and after each workout. If anything causes discomfort or pain, alter the exercise or stop and consult with a trained teacher.

Gradual Progression: As you grow more acquainted with the exercises, gradually increase the intensity, length, or complexity of each movement. This may assist to avoid injuries and maintain continuing improvement.

good Form: Maintain good alignment and posture during each workout. This will allow you to get the most out of your exercise while also lowering the chance of strain or injury.

Rest and Recovery: Give your body time to relax and heal between sessions. Pilates may be done multiple times per week, but you should listen to your body and adapt the frequency as required.

Seek Professional Help: Take courses or work with a trained Pilates teacher, particularly if you're just beginning out. They may give you tailored advice, correct your form, and help you advance securely.

As a beginner, you may have a safe and successful Pilates practice by dividing your workout into a warm-up, major exercises, and cool-down, and advancing gradually while listening to your body and seeking expert coaching.

CHAPTER THREE

Common Mistakes Beginners Make in Pilates

Lack of Core Engagement: Failure to correctly engage the core may cause tension in other muscles and limit the efficacy of activities.

Improper Breathing: Failure to coordinate breathing and movement may break the flow of the workouts and reduce their efficacy.

Excessive arching of the lower back during activity may strain the spine, causing pain or damage.

Poor Posture: Slouching or rounding the shoulders may cause muscular imbalances and tension in the neck and back.

Using Momentum: Performing exercises with momentum rather than controlled, precise motions might impair workout efficacy and increase injury risk.

Tips for Correcting Pilates Form and Technique

Focus on Core Engagement: Before beginning any activity, bring your navel towards your spine to activate your deep abdominal muscles. This will assist to strengthen your core and protect your lower back.

Practice Proper Breathing: Match your breath to your motions, breathing deeply with your nose and expelling thoroughly through your mouth.

Maintain Proper Alignment: Keep your spine neutral, with a natural curvature in your lower back and relaxed shoulders away from your ears.

Move Mindfully: Perform each movement deliberately and with control, emphasizing the quality of your actions above speed or quantity.

Use Props for Support: Blocks, straps, and balls may help you maintain perfect alignment and deepen your stretches without jeopardizing your technique.

Preventing Injury During Pilates Practice

Start Slowly: Begin with simple exercises and progressively increase the intensity and complexity of your workouts as you gain confidence.

Listen to Your Body: If anything causes discomfort or suffering, stop immediately and adapt the activity, or get advice from a certified teacher.

Use Proper Equipment: To avoid mishaps, make sure you're using the correct equipment for each activity and that it's properly set up.

Stay Hydrated: Drink lots of water before, during, and after your exercise to avoid muscular cramps.

Allow your body to rest and heal in between sessions to avoid overuse problems.

As a beginner, you may have a safe and productive Pilates practice by paying attention to these frequent faults and following these guidelines for refining form and technique while avoiding injury.

Transitioning from Beginning to Intermediate Pilates

Increase Intensity: Introduce more difficult workouts that target various muscle groups or need more stability and balance.

Add Props: To add variation and difficulty to your exercises, use props like resistance bands, Pilates balls, or foam rollers.

Focus on Form: Pay special attention to your form and technique to ensure that you are in appropriate alignment and using the right muscles.

Explore Advanced movements: Begin adding advanced Pilates movements, such as the Teaser or the Swan, with the help of a competent teacher.

Listen to Your Body: As you improve, be aware of any discomfort or pain and alter workouts accordingly to prevent damage.

Exploring Various Pilates Styles and Classes

Mat Pilates focuses on movements done on a mat utilizing body weight as resistance. It's an excellent choice for beginners and can be readily tailored to various fitness levels.

Reformer Pilates makes use of a Pilates reformer equipment, which includes a sliding carriage, springs, and straps. It offers additional resistance and a wider range of motion than mat Pilates.

Barre Pilates combines Pilates workouts with ballet and dance aspects, supported by a ballet barre. It aims to improve strength, flexibility, and posture.

Clinical Pilates is often used in rehabilitation settings and is customized to individual requirements, focusing on treating particular areas of weakness or injury.

Setting goals and tracking progress in Pilates

Identify Your Goals: Whether you want to improve core strength, increase flexibility, or reach a certain workout milestone, be clear about what you want to accomplish.

Create a Plan: Create a planned training schedule that includes specific exercises and milestones to help you achieve your objectives.

Track Your Progress: Keep a notebook or use a fitness app to record your exercises and any gains in strength, flexibility, or endurance.

Recognize and celebrate your accomplishments along the road to remain motivated and encouraged to keep growing.

Stay Consistent: Consistency is essential for noticing success in Pilates. Aim to practice often and make tweaks to your strategy as required to keep pushing yourself and moving toward your objectives.

THE END